I0102002

IT'S YOUR LIFE – VITAMINS & SUPPLEMENTS FOR ALL AGES

Professor Norman Ratcliffe

Copyright © 2012 by Professor Norman Ratcliffe

All rights reserved. This book, or parts thereof,
may not be reproduced in any form without
permission.

*A catalogue record for this book is available
from the British Library*

ISBN: 978-1-907962-61-5

Published by Cranmore Publications

www.cranmorepublications.co.uk

This book is dedicated to my parents whose undying faith in my academic capabilities allowed me to pursue a scientific career. My gratitude also goes to my sister, Teri King, whose success as an author and constant encouragement and advice were such sources of inspiration. Thanks too to my many friends for tolerating so many mealtime discussions on health and diet as well as the unsolicited advice given to them!

Finally, I wish to thank Dr. Duncan McLaren of Swansea Metropolitan University for his outstanding enthusiasm and imagination during creation of sections of this book as well as Doreen Montgomery of Rupert Crew Ltd for her patient and helpful comments of the manuscript.

"IT'S YOUR LIFE"

THE AUTHOR

- **Professor Norman Ratcliffe** is a founder member of a team that recently discovered a new antibiotic potentially capable of curing MRSA and *Clostridium difficile*. This work was presented to Prince Phillip at St. James's Palace, London and was the subject of major media attention in the UK on ITV News and in many leading newspapers, including the Wall Street Journal, around the World. He is a Fellow of the Royal Society of Medicine and has previously run a "Health Alert" blood-testing company. He has published over 200 books and research papers on immunology, cancer invasion, influenza, tropical diseases and MRSA. He played squash for Wales, ran the London Marathon at the age of 50 and works-out regularly in the gym.

- **Professor Ratcliffe** retired recently after 25 years as a University Research Professor. He decided to finally complete "It's Your Life" after 5 years work in order to help the many people who are confused about health and fitness issues and who have constantly been asking his advice.

"IT'S YOUR LIFE"

THE SERIES

Professor Norman Ratcliffe's comprehensive book on health is: *It's Your Life: End the confusion from inconsistent health advice:*

www.cranmorepublications.co.uk/6

This book will often be referred to as IYL. Alongside this comprehensive book there is a series of smaller *It's Your Life: End the confusion from inconsistent health advice* books; this book is the fourth in the series. The aim of the series is to give advice to people in specific areas; all of the areas covered in the series are also included in IYL. The series is as follows:

It's Your Life – A Healthy Diet Made Easy

www.cranmorepublications.co.uk/61

It's Your Life – Avoiding Harmful Chemicals in Your Food

www.cranmorepublications.co.uk/62

It's Your Life – Avoid the Cocktail Effect of Harmful Chemicals in Your Body

www.cranmorepublications.co.uk/63

It's Your Life – Vitamins and Supplements For All Ages

www.cranmorepublications.co.uk/64

It's Your Life – Exercise For All Ages

www.cranmorepublications.co.uk/65

The main advice arising from IYL has also been summarised in:

117 Health Tips: A quick guide for a healthy life

www.cranmorepublications.co.uk/7

Contents

Chapter 1   **13**

Vitamins and supplements 1 – take or not to take?

   confusion from conflicting media reports

   effect of food processing on vitamins and minerals

   need for vitamin and mineral supplements

   tables and functions of vitamins and minerals

Chapter 2   **69**

Vitamins and supplements 2 - the bottom line

why the majority of the UK population need
supplements

what to take explained

detailed recommendations for specific groups of people:

normal people, pregnant and menopausal women,

babies, children, seniors, drinkers, smokers, diabetics,

vegetarians and obese people included

Reference sources for conclusions   **146**

CHAPTER 1

VITAMINS AND SUPPLEMENTS - 1

THE "TAKE OR NOT TAKE" DILEMMA

i.   What evidence indicates the need for vitamins and supplements?

ii. What "goodness" is left in our food after processing?

iii. Tables of vitamins and supplements including functions and doses.

"To Take Or Not To Take That Is The Question?"

ARE YOU CONFUSED as to whether or not to take supplements? No wonder, just look at some of the news headlines that have appeared and have done much to add to our confusion:

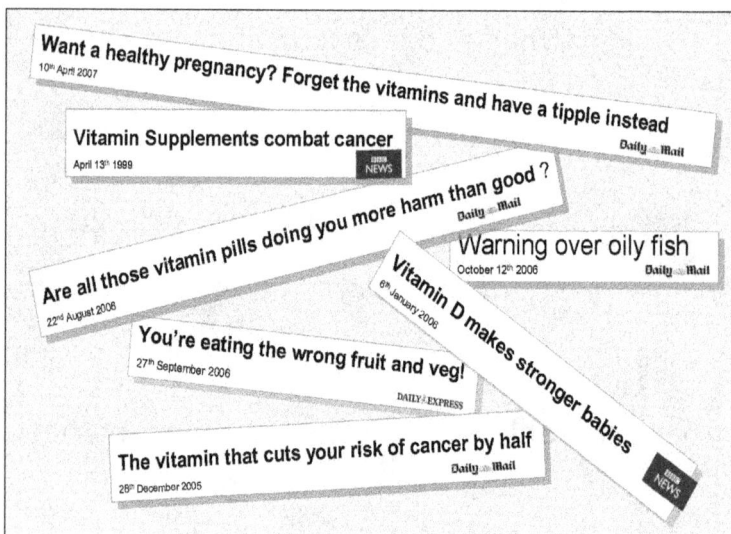

Want a healthy pregnancy? Forget the vitamins and have a tipple instead
10th April 2007
Daily Mail

Vitamin Supplements combat cancer
April 13th 1999
BBC NEWS

Are all those vitamin pills doing you more harm than good?
Daily Mail
22nd August 2006

Warning over oily fish
October 12th 2006
Daily Mail

Vitamin D makes stronger babies
6th January 2006
BBC NEWS

You're eating the wrong fruit and veg!
27th September 2006
DAILY EXPRESS

The vitamin that cuts your risk of cancer by half
28th December 2005
Daily Mail

Many such articles appear almost daily in newspapers, magazines and books **advocating the use of dietary supplements** while doctors and many nutritionists recommend obtaining all necessary vitamins and minerals from a **"healthy balanced diet"**.

What exactly is a "healthy balanced diet"?

As described in Chapter 1 of IYL (pages 26-28), a balanced diet would include a combination of foods from all the main food groups (below) at each meal. Thus, in theory, the balanced diet should provide all our daily requirements of vitamins and minerals.

1. **Bread, cereals, pasta, rice or potatoes** i.e., high in carbohydrate or "starchy" foods.

2. **Fruit and vegetables** (at least 5 per portions per day – see Chapter 1 of IYL) for healthy carbohydrate, protein (pulses), fibre and vitamins.

3. **Meat as a source of protein** to include red meat, poultry, fish, eggs, or meat substitutes such as nuts and pulses (peas, beans and lentils). Avoid too much red meat (beef, pork, ham, lamb) i.e. not every day.

4. **Milk and dairy products** to include milk, cheese and yoghurt (all low-fat or skimmed) to provide some protein but also calcium and B vitamins.

THERE ARE, HOWEVER, SEVERAL PROBLEMS:

- How do we know if our food contains all the vitamins and minerals that we require?

- We tend to have too little time for selecting the food we eat.

- Obesity levels in the UK are soaring with over 12 million adults projected to be obese by 2010. The UK is now the obesity capital of Europe.

- There are about 3 million people in the UK suffering from malnutrition.

CONCLUSIONS

1. Obviously, a huge number of people in the UK do not have a balanced diet. It is therefore unhelpful for the medical experts to repeatedly advise that "vitamin and mineral supplements are not required if you have a balanced diet".

2. Processed or convenience foods are the main culprits responsible for producing obesity and poorly balanced diets. There is also concern over the poor diet of 15-21 year olds, many of whom are also at risk of malnutrition (see reference 76). In addition, of the estimated 3 million malnourished people in the UK, a large number are **elderly and are at particular risk in care homes and hospitals** (see reference 77).

There is also concern about:

THE NUTRITIONAL VALUE OF OUR FOOD

- Even if we adopt an apparently balanced diet what guarantee do we have that our food is providing all the essential vitamins and minerals required?

- Problems with the nutritional content of our food have been highlighted for some years but mainly ignored. Joanne Blythman has researched this topic extensively in her books entitled "The Food We Eat" (1996) and "Bad Food Britain" (2006) (references 78, 79).

- Basically, as a Nation, we shop for food in supermarkets due to time constraints and the convenience of finding everything we need in one location. The problem is that as a result we are hooked on convenience foods that are often **highly processed with their nutritional value degraded**.

- It is true that the supermarkets stock "fresh" fruit and vegetables but many of these are foreign in origin and harvested days or weeks previously with the loss of vital vitamins and minerals. Apparently, **our food may now be "nutritionally impoverished"** (Blythman, 2006, reference 79).

WHAT IS FOOD PROCESSING?

This includes all the stages the food goes through before it is eaten. Processing thus involves the treatment during growing such as spraying with pesticides, as well as special techniques that the food subsequently goes through before eating including milling, preservation, storage, transportation and cooking, all of which will partially degrade the vitamin and mineral content of the food.

a. Growing - Conventional Farming Versus Organic Farming

- Most of our food crops are grown by intensive farming with the aid of synthetic fertilizers. According to the **Food Standards Agency** (FSA), the **nutritional content of these foods is no less** than crops grown organically (see reference 80). The FSA was set up by the Government to protect public health in relation to food.

- **The FSA's conclusion contrasts the view of the Soil Association** (SA), a charitable organization independent of Government and concerned with promoting organic food and farming, which concluded (see reference 81) that organic food had higher levels of vitamin C, as well as of other antioxidants and essential minerals.

- The SA's conclusion was based on a review of 41 studies from around the World and included evidence that between the years of 1941 and 1991, trace elements (=dietary components, such as copper, iron, selenium, and zinc, present only in minute quantities in our food but essential for maintaining health, see Table 2, below) **in conventionally grown fruit and vegetables had fallen by 76%.**

- Clearly, the debate concerning the nutritional values of conventional versus organically grown foods has some way to run and requires more scientific examination. Unfortunately, the FSA's view may be questioned as it is a Government related agency (remember BSE and the "healthy hamburger") while the SA, it could also be argued, is also biased in favour of organic food.

- **Recently, however, a 18 million euros, EU-funded project, showed that organic vegetables (including potatoes, carrots, cabbage and lettuce) and fruit contain up to 40 percent more antioxidants (such as vitamin C) than conventionally-farmed produce. Organic milk was also found to contain 60 percent more antioxidants (such as vitamin E) and beneficial fatty** acids, including omega 3. In addition, organic food was shown to contain lower levels of pesticides and heavy metals. The research was included in the EU "Quality Low Imput Food (QLIF)" project and lead by Professor Carlo Leifert. The research involved over 31 institutes, companies and universities and took place over 5 years from March 2004 to April 2009. Most important too was the fact that to achieve these results good agricultural practices were required and details of these were included in the reports (See, www.qlif.org for leaflets and links).

- Controversially, the FSA commissioned a report on organic versus conventionally produced food, published in 2009, which concluded that although differences exist between these foods, they were "not large enough to be of any public health significance" (see references 82, 83). The FSA study seems to have ignored the Leifert reports (www.qlif.org) although details were being released of these in 2007.

WHO SHOULD THE POOR CONFUSED PUBLIC BELIEVE?

- The FSA report was not an original experimental study but a review of previously published work. The analyses included the results from studies published several decades ago probably before the best agricultural practices had been developed for organic food. The importance of such best practice was emphasized by Leifert and colleagues (see, www.qlif.org).

- In contrast to the FSA review, the Leifert QLIF reports were based on large scale, original experimental studies actually growing crops and rearing animals under optimised conventional and organic conditions.

- There has been widespread criticism of the FSA report for ignoring the QLIF reports.

- Until the FSA considers the QLIF reports objectively and gives reasons for rejecting such important research, then it is logical to accept the findings of the extremely comprehensive QLIF study.

- In addition, most importantly, **many people buy organic food not because of nutritional**

advantages, but because of the lower levels of pesticide residues in organic food. The FSA even supports this point of view.

Many people already believe that organic food:

Tastes better

Has increased nutrient content

Undoubtedly has reduced contamination with pesticides

Has environmental benefits that preserve and encourage wildlife as a result of the use of fewer chemicals and intercropping

Other people point out that with organic food:

Carbon emissions may be much higher as so much is imported

Since yields are lower, more land is required for growing crops

There are reports, for example in chickens, that organic food has higher contamination rates with harmful microorganisms

If you decide to opt for organic food then do this very selectively (see Chapter 4 of IYL for details of which organic foods to choose) to avoid wasting money.

b. Growing - Use of Pesticides

This is, of course, part of the growing process but deserves some separate consideration due to the possible involvement of pesticide residues in the development of human disease. There is now evidence to show that about 30% of our basic conventionally grown foods contain pesticide residues (see Tables 1 to 3 in Chapter 4 of IYL) but the effect of these residues on our health is debatable (discussed in detail in Chapter 6 of IYL). Two things, however, are clear:

i. Our bodies contain cocktails of chemical pollutants derived from pesticides in our food, from worming agents in our livestock, from chemicals contaminating the air we breathe and from products we use on our bodies or in our homes (see details in Chapter 6 of IYL "The Cocktail Effect"). These chemicals may interact in the body to compromise our health.

ii. We must not, due to our fear of chemical contamination, **completely stop eating** vegetables and fruit grown conventionally. The benefits of the "five a day" policy must far outweigh the harm resulting from a diet free of vegetables and fruit. Again, refer to Chapter 4 of IYL "Is Our Food Safe?" for selecting foods with the lowest pesticide contamination levels.

c. Milling – OUR OBSESSION WITH WHITE BREAD AND RICE

- White flour and white rice are made by **removing the outer layers of the wheat or rice seeds** using special milling machines. This produces the white flour for making white bread and pasta, as well as the polished white rice that most people buy.

- We have been brainwashed into thinking that anything white is superior and healthy but this is simply not true. **The outer layers of the wheat and rice seeds contain over 90% of the bran and most of the vitamins and minerals.**

Figure 1. Showing wholemeal and white loaves and the possible advantages and disadvantages of eating each type of bread

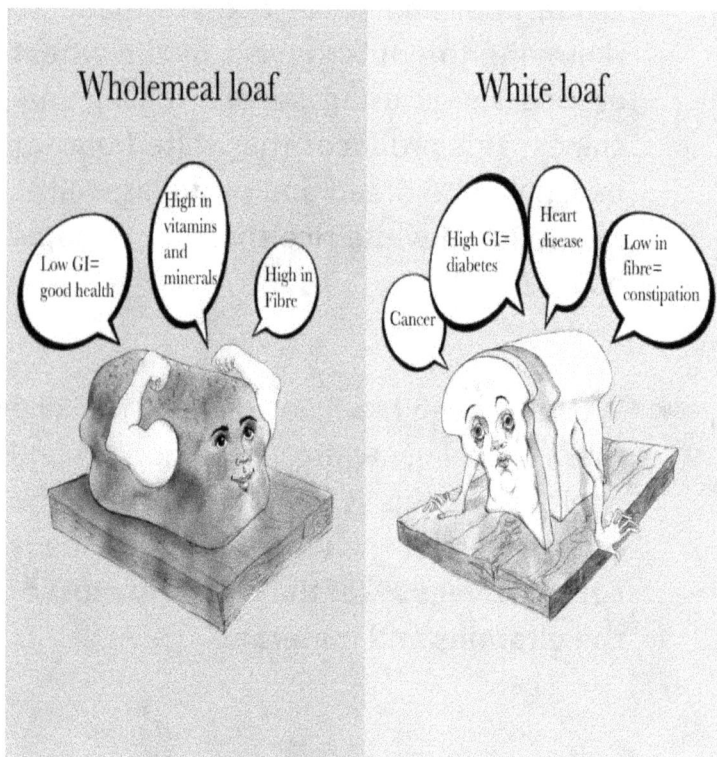

- Generally speaking, white flour is worse for us than white rice simply because white flour is also subjected to **bleaching with toxic chemicals**.

- **Thus, white flour is devoid of essential nutrients and is usually eaten by people who subsequently suffer with higher rates of heart disease, some cancers and type II diabetes (i.e. not dependent on insulin injections but treated by diet and exercise, see reference 84, for example).**

- Just think of the number of biscuits and cakes on the supermarket shelves that have been made with white flour. Even white bread "fortified" with added synthetic vitamins and nutrients is not nearly as good as bread (organic) made from wholemeal or whole grains. White rice, however, does still contain some protein, vitamins and minerals.

33

Figure2. Wholemeal and whole grain loaves

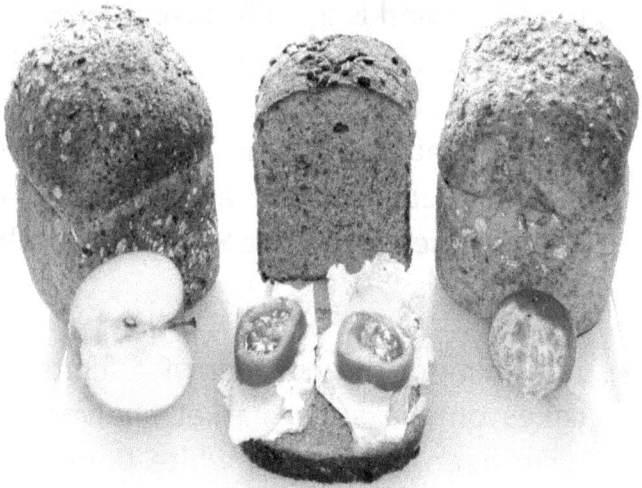

d. Preservation and Storage

These are necessary in order to prevent break-down of the food by microbes and enzymes so it can be stored and transported before use. There are many preservation techniques and the main advantages and disadvantages of the various methods are shown below in Table 1.

Table 1. ADVANTAGES AND DISADVANTAGES OF MAIN METHODS USED TO PRESERVE FOOD

Preservation method	Advantages	Disadvantages
Refrigeration and freezing	Good for nutrient preservation	Slow loss of nutrients, blanching reduces levels of some vitamins

Canning (tinned food)	Food can be stored at room temperature for long periods	Loss of water-soluble nutrients eg. vitamin C, riboflavin, thiamine into canning fluid
Smoking and curing mainly of meat and fish	Dries, flavours and preserves food	Smoked food may be linked to stomach and other cancers
Drying mainly of fruits, meats, fish, cereals, soup, coffee	Removes water prevents microbial growth and stops enzymes that breakdown food	Sulphites sometimes added to dried fruit may cause allergies. Limited loss of vitamin B and C

Chemical additives includes nitrites, nitrates, sulphur dioxide, benzoates etc.	Improves shelf life, appearance and taste of food and inhibits microbial growth and poisoning	Linked to cancer formation, allergies, fertility problems, and adverse children's behavior – see Chapters 5 and 6 of IYL
Heat sterilisation of milk and juices (pasteurization and ultra-heat treatment, UHT)	Long shelf life at room temperature	Loss of some nutrients but less than in in canning

Added salt or sugar eg. meats and jams	Good for nutrient preservation	High salt content associated with high blood pressure
Irradiation of limited use and mainly for spices and condiments in UK	Prolongs shelf life, killing insects and bacteria, delays fruit ripening and sprouting in vegetables	Some safety concerns and loss of nutrients including antioxidants*

* See details in reference 85

THE CONCLUSION from Table 1, above, is that all preservation methods either result in the loss of vitamins or minerals or else may result in concerns about health safety. Obviously, for maximizing our intake of vitamins and minerals, we should all be eating recently harvested/killed foodstuffs. In our modern, fast-paced, society this is clearly impossible all the time. The secret is to compromise and be aware of the shortcomings of the modern diet and whenever possible to introduce locally grown, fresh food. Failing this, then frozen foods are acceptable with limited nutrient loss and few if any chemical additives.

e. Food Transportation

- Transportation of food leads to a **significant loss of vital nutrients**, the extent of which will depend upon the time and distance travelled. In the USA, it has been estimated that the components of a basic meal have travelled 1500 miles to arrive at the dinner plate.

- Many of the numerous fruits and vegetables on display in supermarkets throughout the year in the UK have also travelled thousands of miles to arrive on the shelves.

- In addition, with green vegetables, the entire marketing route from harvesting, blanching, freezing, transportation, storage, distribution, purchase and consumption has been estimated to take about 60 days (see reference 86). During this time, spinach, beans and peas all lose significant amounts of vitamin C, which reaches more than a 50 percent loss with spinach.

- Remember much organic produce is also imported and has thus undergone significant nutrient loss thus cancelling out one important benefit, i.e. higher vitamin content, of buying organic food.

- Locally purchased, non-organic, fruit and vegetables will probably match organic produce for nutrient content although the other benefits of organic, such as reduced pesticide contamination, will still apply. The optimum is to buy locally grown organic food, not only for the nutritional advantages, but also to reduce the carbon emissions from transportation which results in global warming.

f. Cooking

Inevitably, cooking food leads to a further loss of nutrients but this will depend upon:

- **The method of cooking** with boiling in excess hot water leading to the loss of many water-soluble vitamins such as vitamins B and C and minerals including calcium. A study on the effect of different cooking methods on the antioxidant content of freshly picked broccoli showed that microwaving, boiling and pressure cooking resulted in 47 to 97 percent loss of antioxidants while **steamed broccoli was similar to the raw vegetable in antioxidant content** (see reference 87). Microwaving, however, was shown by the same authors to be far less damaging to the nutrient content of vegetables if the amount of water used for cooking was kept to a minimum.

- **The temperature and the length of the cooking time** which if too high/long will result in further nutrient loss. This is particularly a problem in cafeterias where food is often kept hot for too long under bright lights.

- **The type of food cooked** with, for example, rice rapidly losing vitamins and minerals unless washed and cooked in minimal volumes of water. In contrast, eggs lose few nutrients during cooking.

- **The nutrient involved** with water-soluble vitamins B and C rapidly lost by boiling while fat-soluble vitamins such as vitamin A are more resistant to leaching into the cooking water.

THE BASIC RULES FOR RETAINING THE MAXIMAL NUTRIENT CONTENT OF FOOD DURING COOKING ARE:

1. Steam food for the minimal time

2. If you boil or microwave then cover the food to retain the steam and speed up the cooking process

3. Use the minimal water for cooking, especially for rice

4. Use the cooking or steaming water as a stock for sauces and stews

5. Do not soak food before cooking i.e. do not prepare the vegetables the previous day and store in water

6. Do not keep the cooked food hot for long but eat as soon as possible

7. Eat some freshly prepared uncooked fruit/vegetables every day

COOKING – IT'S NOT ALL BAD NEWS

Cooking not only makes food more palatable but also kills off harmful microbes. In addition, it releases from the cells of fruit and vegetables higher concentrations of antioxidants such as lycopene for absorption in the gut. Lycopene has multiple benefits in preventing prostate cancer and cardiovascular disease (see Chapter 1 of IYL).

WHAT IS THE EVIDENCE THAT WE NEED TO TAKE
VITAMINS AND OTHER SUPPLEMENTS?

1. From the section above on food processing, it is obvious that in many cases there may be serious depletion of essential nutrients, such as vitamins and minerals in food.

2. Recent studies do indicate that certain key nutrients are at too low levels in our diet.

3. We also know that there are about 3 million people, many of whom are elderly, suffering malnutrition in the UK. Most of these would probably benefit from supplements.

4. Research has also shown that many people have levels of vitamins in their bodies below recommended daily allowances. This topic will be discussed in Chapter 2 in detail after we have briefly listed, below (Tables 2 and 3), the main vitamins and minerals required in our diet.

Don't just plough through these Tables as they are for your reference after you have decided which supplements you need to take (see Chapter 2 "The Bottom Line")

Table 2.   FUNCTIONS AND SOURCES OF VITAMINS THAT ARE COMMONLY TAKEN AS DIETARY SUPPLEMENTS

Name ↓	RDA[1] + Deficiency Symptoms	Safe Upper Limit [2] Per day	In Which Foods	Functions to Maintain
Vitamin A (retinol, beta carotene)	0.6-0.7mg[3] Night blindness; other problems in developing countries	General use as supplement not advised, especially by smokers	Liver and fish oils, yellow /orange fruit and vegetables, leafy greens	Healthy bones, teeth, hair, eyesight, and lining of mouth, nose, lungs and reproductive system

Vitamin B1 (thiamine)	1.1-1.5 mg[3] Muscular weakness, tiredness, poor memory; alcoholics often affected	Unknown, 40 mg+?	Offal, lean meat, fish, eggs, milk, whole grain bread, cereals and pasta, brown rice	Energy release from food; brain, nerve and heart functions; prevents brain damage in alcoholics
Vitamin B2 (riboflavin)	1.1-1.3 mg[3] Sores around nose and lips; itching, sore throat; sensitivity to light	Unknown, but no more 40 mg advised	Liver, cheese, eggs, milk, green vegetables like broccoli, whole grain bread, cereals and pasta	Energy release from food; healthy skin, hair, nails, eyesight; assists adrenalin production and iron absorption

Vitamins & Supplements

Vitamin B3 (niacin which occurs as nicotina-mide and nicotinic acid)	13-17 mg[3] Eruptions on skin in sunlight; swollen tongue; insomnia and diarrhoea	Unknown but no more 35-50 mg advised	Liver, red meat, poultry and fish, whole grain bread, cereals, nuts and beans	Energy release from food; healthy skin; promotes nervous system and gut functions and sex hormone production
Vitamin B5 (pantothen-ic acid)	6 mg Deficiency rare and only seen with severe starvation; burning feet and restless-ness	Unknown but no more 500 mg advised	Liver, kidney, chicken, beef, eggs, broccoli, whole grain bread and cereals, nuts and beans	Energy release from food; essential for growth and healthy nervous system; synthesis of hormones, red blood cells and antibodies

Vitamin B6 (pyridoxine)	No RDA but 1.2-1.6 mg^3 advised Deficiency unusual; signs are dermatitis, sore tongue, anaemia, confusion, irritability, impaired immunity	10 mg	Liver, chicken, red meat, whole grain bread and cereals, avocadoes, bananas, tuna, salmon, sunflower seeds, peanut butter	Red blood cells and haemoglobin synthesis, immune and nervous system functions, normal levels of blood sugar, absorption of vitamin B 12, production of some hormones

Vitamin B7 (biotin or vitamin H)	RDA (USA) 0.3 mg (300 µg) Deficiency rare; dermatitis, rash around eyes, exhaustion, loss of appetite, muscle pain	Unknown but no more than 0.9 mg (900 µg) advised	Liver, kidney, milk, cheese, egg yolk, nuts, bananas, broccoli, soya, whole grain bread and cereals	Hair, nails and skin? Also for energy production
Vitamin B9 (folic acid)	0.2-0.4 mg[4] (=200-400 µg) Anaemia; spina bifida in newborn babies	Unknown but no more 1 mg advised	Liver, whole grain bread and cereals, broccoli, spinach, nuts, oranges	Formation of blood cells; healthy nervous system in unborn babies

Vitamin B12 (cobalamin)	1.5 µg Pernicious anaemia, brain, nerve and heart damage	Unknown but no more 2 mg (2000 µg) advised	Animal produce- liver, meat, fish, eggs, milk, but also in soya milk and added to cereals	Formation of red blood cells; healthy nervous system
Vitamin C (ascorbic acid)	40-60 mg^3 Scurvy with bleeding gums, weakness, painful joints, anaemia, and bruising	Unknown, more than 1gram may give gut problems	Citrus fruits i.e. oranges; other fruits such as berries, kiwis; also in green leafy vegetables including spinach and broccoli	Healthy bones, teeth and gums; iron absorption and wound healing; resistance to infection due to antioxidant function

Vitamins & Supplements

Vitamin D (calciferol)	No RDA but 10-15 µg^3 advised Failure of bone growth, and rickets in children	Unknown, but no more than 25 µg advised	Liver, dairy produce, oily fish but main source is sunlight on skin	Healthy teeth, bones, nerves, muscles and blood clotting; may reduce cancer
Vitamin E (tocophe-rol)	No RDA but 3-15 mg (4.5-22.5 IU) advised. Deficiency rare but may result from harmful action of oxygen radicals	Unknown but no more than 540 mg (800 IU) advised	Highest in vegetable oils (olive, sunflower, corn, soya); also in whole grain bread and cereals, meat, leafy greens-spinach and kale	Antioxidant activity, protecting cell membranes from oxygen radicals arising from cell processes and environmen-tal pollution such as cigarette

	from cell processes or pollution such as cigarette smoke			smoke. Prevents anaemia and, although proof incomplete, may slow aging and reduce heart attacks?
Vitamin K (phylloqui-none)	No RDA but 120 µg per day sufficient. Deficiency unusual but may result from gut problems resulting in poor absorption	Unknown but no more than 1 mg advised	Liver, milk and eggs, fatty fish and fish oils, plant oils like soya and rape seed, dark leafy vegetables – spinach and broccoli	Coagulation of blood and healthy bones

1. RDA (Recommended Daily Allowances) **from all sources,** including food, drink and supplements, given for adults 18 yr + only. Children less than 18 yr require significantly lower doses (see references 88, 89).

2. Safe Upper Limit per day (SUL) (see reference 90).

3. The lower RDA is for women and the upper RDA for men.

4. 0.4mg folic acid is recommended as a supplement for pregnant women up to week 12 of pregnancy.

Table 3. FUNCTIONS AND SOURCES OF MINERALS, TRACE METALS AND SOME MISCELLANEOUS FACTORS THAT ARE COMMONLY TAKEN AS DIETARY SUPPLEMENTS

Name ↓	RDA[1] + Deficiency Symptoms	Safe Upper Limit [2] Per day	In Which Foods	Functions to Maintain
Boron	No RDA but 1.5-2 mg advised Osteoporosis in elderly?	6 mg	Nuts, fresh fruit, peas, beans and green vegetables	Healthy bones by preventing osteoporosis and arthritis by influencing calcium and magnesium balance?
Calcium	800 mg[3] Weak bones	1,500 mg	Dairy products, nuts,	Healthy bones and teeth, muscle and

	and teeth, osteoporosis, stunted growth		salmon, sardines, green leafy vegetables like broccoli and cabbage, tofu	heart functions, blood clotting, mental health (?) and may protect against breast, prostate and colon cancers?
Chromium	No RDA but at least 0.025 mg required Deficiency rare outside hospital	Unknown but no more than 10 mg advised. General use not advised	Meat, whole grain bread and cereals, pulses and spices	Insulin levels and thus influences energy obtained from food
Copper	No RDA Anaemia and bone malformation	No more than 10 mg advised	Liver, shellfish, whole grain bread, cereals, nuts	Functions of many enzymes, energy production, growth, immunity, blood cell formation, heart and brain functions

Iodine	150 µg [4] Goiter, lethargy, weakness, weight gain, lower IQ, miscarriage, stillbirth, and birth defects	No more than 500 µg Advised	Milk, cheese, turkey, marine fish, shellfish, sea salt and seaweed (kelp)	Production of thyroid hormones that regulate energy production; also required for development of brain in foetus and children
Iron	8-18 mg [5] Anaemia with associated fatigue and palpitations	Unknown but adverse effects above 50 mg	Liver, red meat, whole grain bread and cereals, oysters, pulses, dark green leafy vegetables, apricots, molasses and tofu	Oxygen transport around body, immune functions and energy production

Magnesium	300-400 mg[5] Deficiency rare but results in fatigue, as well as heart, gut, nervous and skeletal disorders	Unknown but no more than 400 mg Advised	In many foods including high levels in whole grain bread and cereals, green leafy vegetables, nuts, brown rice	Energy production, cell multiplication and cell interactions, vitamin D and hormone activities
Manganese	No RDA but Adequate Dietary Intake set at 2-5 mg for adults. Deficiency rare	Unknown but no more than 0.5 mg as a supplement?	Tea (particular-ly green), whole grain bread and cereals, spinach, pineapple, nuts, brown rice	Enzyme functions involved in many processes such as antioxidant activity, bone and cartilage formation, wound healing, control of blood sugar and cholesterol levels

Phosphorus	700 mg Deficiency rare and at starvation in anorexics and Alcoholics	Unknown but no more than 250 mg as a supplement	Meat, poultry, fish, dairy, whole grain bread and cereals, nuts, beans, peas	Energy production, bone and tissue structure, hormone and enzyme activities
Potassium	No RDA, 3,500 mg recommend-ed Deficiency from vomiting, diarrhoea, alcoholism, sweating, dieting, heart failure resulting in muscle weakness, fatigue, abnormal heart beat	Unknown but no more than 4900 mg	Liver, meat, fish, milk, fruit (bananas, citrus, raisins), vegetables (potatoes, spinach)	Correct internal water balance of cells and tissues that is essential for all life processes

Selenium	55 µg Deficiency in long-term hospitalized patients on artificial diets also in Crohn's disease, causes heart and joint damage	450 µg	Offal, pork, fish, whole grain bread Brazil nuts (very high levels), seeds	Antioxidant activity against harmful free radicals produced by body and may help protect against some cancers?
Sodium **(chloride)**	No RDA but 3-4 g recommend-ed in adults. Deficiency rare except with excess sweating	Unknown but no more than 6 g in diet advised. Not used as supplement	Main source is from processed food and salt added at mealtimes	With potassium, determines correct internal water balance of cells and tissues as well as blood volume and pressure; also component of body secretions

Zinc	15 mg Poor growth and development, reduced immunity and wound healing, mental retardation, nerve damage, night blindness	42 mg	Oysters (very high levels), all meats, milk and cheese, cereals and bread	Immune functioning, growth and development, reproduction, many enzyme functions throughout body
		SOME ADDITIONAL MISCELLANEOUS SUPPLEMENTS[6]		
Aspirin	75mg (coated)	Long term use not advised unless under medical supervision	Pills	Prevention of colon and prostate cancer, heart attacks, strokes and Alzheimer's?

Co-enzyme Q10 (ubiquinone)	No RDA but 50-200 mg advised as supplement depending on disease	Unknown, no toxicity reported	Offal, oily fish, whole grain bread and cereals, peanuts and vegetable oils	Energy production, antioxidant activity, periodontal health
Fish Oils[7] (Omega-3 Fatty Acids)	No RDA but 500-1000 mg capsules usually taken containing 450 mg fatty acids. Capsules vary in content of fatty acids	Unknown, but beware cod liver oil capsules which contain high levels of vitamin A	Omega-3 fatty acids present naturally in fish, also in tofu, and soybeans, walnuts flaxseed and oils made from these but plant sources are of limited use.[7]	Healthy heart, brain development in foetus, and joint motility to reduce symptoms of arthritis. Capsules of fish oil also contain vitamin D (see benefits in Table 2)

Garlic	No RDA but 600-900 mg by mouth recommended	Unknown	In raw cloves, pills, powder, oil, juice syrup or tincture	Reduction of cholesterol levels. Prevention of cancer and infections? Thinning of blood and reduction of blood pressure?
Glucosamine sulphate or hydrochloride	No RDA but 1500 mg by mouth recommended	Unknown but beware of sulphate if blood pressure high	Pills/capsules	Treatment for pain and immobility of osteoarthritis

1. RDA (Recommended Daily Allowances **from all sources including food, drink and supplements**) given mainly for adults 18 yr + only. Children less than 18 yr require significantly lower doses while elderly people and pregnant women may need higher levels (see references 88, 89).

2.   Safe Upper Limit per day (SUL) (see reference 90).

3.   Higher levels of calcium (another 500 mg) may be required in breast-feeding women and additional calcium may be needed by elderly people (see Chapter 2 for details).

4.   Pregnant and breast feeding women may require iodine supplements to raise intake levels but consult your doctor. Multivitamins contain iodine.

5.   The lower iron RDA is for men and the higher RDA is for women.

6.   These supplements are included just as examples of the many other substances taken daily by people. Only garlic and coenzyme Q10 are diet related.

7.   It is better to use fish oil rather than cod liver oil supplements since the latter also have high concentrations of vitamin A which could be toxic to pregnant and elderly people. Pregnant women should also use pure sources of omega-3 such as krill as fish oils may be contaminated with heavy metals and pesticides. Plant sources of omega-3 fatty acids, such as flaxseeds, walnuts and Soya, may not be utilized as efficiently by the body as fish oils but opinions differ (see reference 91).

CHAPTER 2

VITAMINS AND SUPPLEMENTS – 2

"THE BOTTOM LINE"

In the UK population of 61.4 million, 45 million people belong to groups likely to benefit from taking vitamin/mineral supplements

What to take is explained

In a hurry? Just identify below which particular group of people you belong to and read your recommended daily vitamin and mineral supplements.

Tables 2 and 3 in Chapter 1 give sources of these vitamins/minerals in different foods and the total recommended daily allowances (RDA) of those required from food, drink and supplements.

WARNING: Vitamin, mineral and herb supplements may interact with medicines (see page 142, below)

REMEMBER, whenever possible, it is better to modify your diet to obtain your vitamins *naturally*, however, many people are probably more likely to take a vitamin pill than change their diet.

SOME BASIC FACTS ABOUT THE UK POPULATION

The UK population was 61.4 million in 2008 which included 39 million 16-64 year olds of which nearly 50% were overweight (27%) or obese (23%).

The 61.4 million people can approximately be broken down into:

1. 19.6 million 16-64 yr olds of normal weight.*

2. 19.6 million 16-64 yr olds over-weight or obese.

3. 9.9 million over 65 yr old.

4. 12.3 million children less than 16 yr old.

5. 3.9 million 16-64 yr olds (included in groups 1 and 2, above) who smoke and/or drink excessively (a very reserved estimate).

6. About 2 million pregnant or breast feeding women (included in groups 1, 2 and 5 (above).

*Some of these "normal" people will include, vegetarians, dieters, diabetics, anaemia sufferers, and Islamic women, all of whom will require supplements.

From the above, an estimate of the number of UK people likely to benefit from taking vitamin and mineral supplements is approximately 45 million. Only about 16 million adults have a normal weight and, hopefully, a balanced diet.

SUPPLEMENT REQUIREMENTS OF DIFFERENT GROUPS OF PEOPLE

i. "NORMAL" HEALTHY PEOPLE   19-59 YEARS OLD.

The vitamin and mineral supplement market in the UK is worth about £300 million per year. Over 40% of adults take supplements with the 50-65 year olds the highest users (see reference 92). The most commonly taken supplements are cod liver oil and multivitamins. Only 2% of supplement consumers take high dose vitamin/minerals, with vitamin C as the most popular for use. Most experts agree that vitamins in supplements do not have the same effect on the body as vitamins eaten in foods. An apple, for example, not only contains vitamin C but also a complex mixture of other vitamins, antioxidants and phytochemicals which interact in the body. The action of a single supplement on the body taken as a pill in isolation will thus be very different to the mixture of vitamins/minerals in fruits or vegetables. Hence the advice from many dieticians and doctors that "**It is unnecessary for normal healthy people to take supplements as we can obtain all our vitamins/minerals from 'a balanced diet' containing at least 5 portions of fruit and vegetables per day**".

UNFORTUNATELY, according to the Foods Standards Agency National Diet & Nutrition Survey in 2004 (see reference 93), of adults aged 19 to 64, only 13% of men and 15% of women ate 5 or more portions of fruit and vegetables per day. In fact, the 19-24 yr old men and women only consumed 1.3 and 1.8 portions, respectively, in comparison to the 50-64 yr olds where the figures were 3.6 and 3.8 portions. Even more worrying is the fact that in the 19-24 yr group, 45% and 27% of men and women, respectively, ate no fruit at all.

It has been estimated that increasing individual fruit and vegetable intake to at least 5-a-day could reduce coronary heart disease by 31% and ischaemic (the most common form of stroke) stroke by 19%. In addition, for stomach, oesophageal, lung and colorectal cancer, the estimated reductions could be 19%, 20%, 12% and 2%, respectively. However, due to hectic lifestyles, people prefer to have ready processed meals and pop a multivitamin rather than taking the trouble to buy and cook fresh food. **WE**

MUST REALISE that with many adults, in the short term, this situation will be hard to change due to constraints in time, attitude, education and finance. The situation with children is more hopeful due to "5-a-day" campaigns underway focused in schools (see reference 94).

As a "normal" weight, healthy person in the 19-59 yr old group, is it necessary to take supplements and if so which ones? The answer will depend upon:

1. Your present diet

2. Your exposure to sunlight

1. Diet – If you are one of the 13% men and 15% women who eat at least 5 fruit or vegetables per day and have a well balanced diet then you may only require vitamin D (see 2. below). There is, however, as discussed in Chapter 1, no guarantee that your "well balanced" diet will contain all your daily requirements of vitamins/minerals due to loss of nutrients during food processing with the use of pesticides or poor storage and over cooking.

2. Exposure to sunlight – It is very difficult to obtain adequate requirements of vitamin D from the diet alone as exposure to sunlight is required for the body to make this vitamin. Indeed, it has been shown that of middle aged British adults, 60% are vitamin D deficient and this is particularly a problem during spring and winter when it may reach 90% (see reference 95).

In addition, you are likely to be very deficient in vitamin D if you are:

a. Asian, Afro-Caribbean or Middle East in origin with very dark skin.

b. Cover the skin through religious or health reasons.

c. Rarely go outside the house (disabled or elderly).

d. Do not eat much meat, oily fish or dairy products.

e. Live in Scotland, Wales or other regions of the UK with little sunshine especially in the poor "summers" of 2007 and 2008.

Exposure of face, legs, arms etc to the sun for 10-15 minutes per day, 2-3 times per week without sunscreen (but with no burning), is recommended so the skin can make sufficient quantities of vitamin D_3 (the most beneficial kind). The body cannot over-produce vitamin D following excessive sun exposure. In addition, vitamin D produced can be stored so that intermittent sun exposure is fine.

In the UK, some foods, such as oily fish, naturally contain vitamin D while others have vitamins/minerals added (fortified). For example, margarine and reduced fat spreads have vitamin D added by law. The amount added, however, is only sufficient to match the levels found naturally in butter and **will not provide the shortfall arising from lack of exposure to the sun.** In addition, many breakfast cereals are also fortified with vitamins D and generally provide about 13% of adult vitamin D daily intake.

> *Despite this fortification, vitamin D deficiency in the UK is rife and the case for taking vitamin D supplements is extremely strong for the normal population as well as for the special groups of people identified below.*

WHY HAVE I FOCUSED ON VITAMIN D SUPPLEMENTATION? Much recent research indicates that adequate intake of vitamin D helps to protect against:

a. Cancers, including breast, prostate and colon

b. Diabetes

c. Problems with thinning of the bones (osteoporosis) resulting in falls and fractures in older, especially menopausal, females (see "Menopausal Women" and "People Over 50-60 yr" groups, below).

What other supplements are regularly taken by this group of 19-59 year old healthy people? These include:

a. Cod liver oil

b. Multivitamins

c. The antioxidant vitamins – A, C, E and selenium

d. Vitamin B

e. Calcium

f. Glucosamine

a. COD LIVER OIL OR FISH OILS for Omega-3 Fatty Acids. Many people take fish oil capsules regularly (1000 mg per day) to maintain and improve joint flexibility and relieve arthritic pain. In addition, fish oils may have many other benefits such as reducing the risk of heart disease, strokes and cancer and maintaining a healthy brain. Again, unfortunately, scientific opinion differs as to the benefits of taking fish oils although the weight of evidence does seem favorable (see reference 96). Taking omega-3 fish oils, which are present naturally in sardines, mackerel, herrings and salmon, in capsules is harmless and can therefore be recommended. Alternatively, eat 2 to 4 portions of oily fish per week such as tinned or fresh mackerel, salmon, trout, herrings, pilchards, kippers, anchovies, tuna (no more than 2 tuna steaks per week) and sardines, all of which contain natural omega-3 oils. Unfortunately, dioxins and mercury are pollutants that may be present at high levels in some oily fish such as shark, marlin, swordfish and types of fresh tuna and should be avoided by pregnant women (see reference 97). **Cod liver oil should be avoided by pregnant women and elderly people as it contains high vitamin A levels (see below). Also, see Chapter 1, Table 3, for correct sources of omega-3 fatty acids.**

b. MULTIVITAMINS are taken by large numbers of people in the belief that they will prevent heart disease, cancer and maintain general health and well-being. For normal people with balanced diets, including 5-a-day fruit or vegetables, there is very little evidence that multivitamins are beneficial in preventing disease. Thus, in 2006, the National Institute of Health (USA) concluded that there is insufficient evidence "to recommend either for or against the use of Multivitamin/Mineral Supplements to prevent chronic disease" (see reference 98). Unfortunately, few studies of multivitamins have been made although some reduction in cancer incidence has been reported (see references 99, 100). However, for many groups of people, including the over 50-60s, the obese, heavy drinkers and smokers (see below) with poor diets, multivitamins will probably be vital for filling gaps in their nutrition. **Most important is the fact that daily multivitamins appear to be safe as long as you check that they contain no more than the recommended daily allowance (=100% of RDA given in Tables 2 & 3, Chapter 1) for the component vitamins and minerals and ONLY TAKE ONE PER DAY.** The following Table 1 will allow you to confirm that your choice of multivitamin does not contain higher than recommended levels of supplements. It also indicates which supplements have been identified by the Foods Standards Agency (see reference 101) as causing side effects in excessive doses above the SUL (Safe Upper Limits as given in Tables 2 & 3, Chapter 1).

Table 1. ADVICE TO CONSUMERS AND MANUFACTURERS ON UPPER THRESHOLD LEVELS OF SUPPLEMENTS*

Nutrient ↓	Threshold triggering advice	Advice of possible side effects
Calcium	More than 1500 mg	This amount of Calcium may cause mild stomach upset in sensitive people.
Iron	More than 20 mg	This amount of Iron may cause mild stomach upset in sensitive people.
Magnesium	More than 400 mg	This amount of Magnesium may cause mild stomach upset in sensitive people.
Manganese	More than 0.5 mg	Long term intake of this amount of Manganese may lead to muscle pain and fatigue.

Nickel	All nickel-containing products	Nickel may cause a skin rash in sensitive people.
Phosphorus	More than 250 mg	This amount of Phosphorus may cause mild stomach upsets in sensitive individuals".
Vitamin A (retinol, beta carotene)	More than 7 mg	Beta carotene may increase the risk of lung cancer in heavy smokers.
Vitamin B3 (niacin= nicotinic acid or nicotina-mide)	More than 20 mg	Better as Nicotinamide form in supplement. If Nicotinic acid is used then this amount may cause skin flushes in sensitive people.
Vitamin B6	More than 10 mg	Long term intakes of this amount of vitamin B6 may lead to mild tingling and numbness. However, safe levels up to 100 mg have been advocated by many medical experts since excess is readily excreted from the body. Do not use high dosage without medical consultation.

| Vitamin C | More than 1000 mg | This amount of Vitamin C may cause mild stomach upset in sensitive people. |
| Zinc | More than 25 mg | Long term intake of this amount of Zinc may lead to anaemia. |

* See reference 101

The percentage RDA (recommended daily allowance) for each component is written on the multivitamin label. There are large numbers of different makes of multivitamins, for example, for children, the over 50s or pregnant women, so make sure you use the appropriate one and avoid excess of vitamin A or beta carotene (no more than 0.6-0.7 mg = 600-700 micrograms = 1998-2331 IU). BEWARE, AS OVER 50% OF MULTIVITAMINS MAY CONTAIN EXCESS VITAMIN A. A US study in 2000 of over 4500 female doctors showed that about 50% took a multivitamin-mineral supplement which is reassuring!

c. THE ANTIOXIDANT VITAMINS include A, C, E and selenium and are taken every day by millions of people in the UK, either in multivitamins or separately at higher doses. These antioxidants have been widely promoted as preventing many diseases such as cancer, heart problems and strokes as well as slowing down the aging process and halting Alzheimer's. This hype was based on the fact that antioxidants neutralise harmful oxygen radicals produced in the body as a result of many cellular activities associated with the utilisation of the oxygen that we breathe. These oxygen radicals then not only kill cells but also attack the DNA and cause mutations leading to aging, cancer and other diseases. **Many people became hooked on vitamin C in the 1970s as a result of:**

1. Professor Linus Pauling, a famous, 20th century, double Nobel Prize winning scientist, who advocated taking mega-doses (10-12 g daily!) of vitamin C for the prevention of the common cold, cardiovascular and other diseases (see reference 102)

2. Media hype of the benefits of antioxidants resulting from research publications on, for example, fruit flies and mice in which scientists engineered animals producing extra amounts of antioxidants in their bodies. The flies lived as much as 30% longer and the mice nearly 20% longer than animals producing normal levels of antioxidants (see references 103, 104). Thus, in theory, we could all live beyond 100 yr old!

However, in the last few years, a number of high profile scientific reviews and organisations have questioned the effectiveness of antioxidant supplements in preventing disease. For example, the British Heart Foundation, (2002), the American Heart Association (2003), and the Foods Standards Agency (2003) have all stated that there is insufficient evidence to recommend taking antioxidants for the prevention or treatment of cancer or cardiovascular disease and advised against their use. A few reviews, including the Cochrane Review (2008) on antioxidants, have even indicated that high doses of antioxidants may be harmful (see reference 105). Needless to say, the media went wild and their headlines irresponsibly shouted out loud that all vitamins were dangerous! Thus, statements such as "Vitamin pill danger", "Vitamins could shorten lifespan" and "Vitamin tablets may do more harm than good" were splashed around everywhere. The end result is that the poor old public are totally confused as to whether taking vitamins is beneficial or harmful to health.

THE TRUTH OF THE MATTER IS THAT:

1. The majority of vitamins (including A, C, E and selenium) are safe provided that the recommended SULs (Safe Upper Limits) are not exceeded (see reference 101). These SULs are given in Tables 2 and 3 of Chapter 1. The reports of harmful effects are worth noting **but most negative reports are reviews** rather than original trials. Thus, the Cochrane Review (see reference 105) added together and then analysed the results of 67 previous clinical trials most of which used different doses and combinations of supplements as well as variable time scales and both healthy and sick patients. **Overall there was little evidence of increased risk of death from taking beta carotene or vitamins A, C, E or selenium** (see, however, "cigarette smokers", page 120 below). However, when the analytical technique was changed and the different antioxidants looked at separately there was a slight significant increase in risk of death with beta carotene (16% increase) and vitamins A (7%) and E (4%) but no increases for vitamin C or selenium. This is all very confusing and the techniques used unsatisfactory with the authors themselves concluding that further research was required.

2. Only you can decide whether you belong to the normal weight, healthy group of people eating at least 5-a-day fruit or vegetables and therefore do or do not require any antioxidant supplements.

3. Most healthy people in the 19-59 age group can obtain any additional antioxidant requirements from a one per day good multivitamin tablet.

4. If you decide to take higher levels of individual antioxidant   supplements (rarely recommended as evidence is mounting as to possible harmful effects) then it would be wise NOT to take a multivitamin as well and to limit yourself to:

   - Beta carotene/vitamin A - better not to supplement at all, especially smokers, pregnant women and the elderly

   - Vitamin C – no more than 250-500 mg/day

   - Vitamin E – no more than 200 IU (134mg) per day

   - Selenium – no more than 350-400 µg per day

5. Whatever you do, avoid advice from websites and magazines which are sponsored or linked to supplement manufacturers, otherwise you will end up spending a fortune on supplements that are unnecessary.

d. VITAMIN B SUPPLEMENTATION The need for vitamin B supplements by the healthy 19-59 yr olds is the subject of debate. Vitamin B is, however, recommended for many other groups of people including pregnant women, the elderly, drinkers, smokers and diabetics (see below).

There is some evidence for vitamin deficiency in healthy adults. For example, it was reported in 2000 that low levels of blood vitamin B-12 are present not only in 17% of the elderly (over 65 yr old) but also in a similar level of 26-64 yr old adults (see reference 106). In addition, about 3 million people in the UK take 100-200mg of vitamin B-6 daily for PMS (pre-menstrual stress), morning sickness or stress. Experimental evidence that high-dosage B6 alleviates this problem is disputed so maybe the effect produced is psychological (the placebo effect). The **patient's belief** that vitamin B-6 will improve their condition may bring about changes in body chemistry triggering the reduction in symptoms obtained.

There is also evidence that the B vitamins (folic acid = vitamin B-9, as well as B-6 and B-12), may help to break down an amino acid in the blood called homocysteine. High homocysteine levels have been linked to heart disease and strokes by promoting the formation of fatty deposits in the arteries and blood clot formation. Much research has been undertaken to prove the role of homocysteine in cardiovascular disease. To date, although heart patients have raised levels of homocysteine, its exact role in heart disease is unknown (see, however, reference 107). Lowering homocysteine by increasing folic acid (B-9), B-6 and B-12 intakes have been advocated to reduce the risk of heart disease.

Increased vitamin B intake can be obtained directly from the diet with 5-a-day fruit and vegetables (see Table 2, Chapter 1) and from vitamin fortified breakfast cereals and bread. Again, if you avoid breakfast cereals or bread and fail to eat sufficient fruit and vegetables then a vitamin supplement will be required. A multivitamin should contain at least 400 micrograms of folic acid but optimal levels of B-6 and B-12 have not been determined. Daily doses of 12.5 mg for B-6 and 500 micrograms for B-12 are safe as long as they do not interact with other drugs being taken. Each of these B vitamins, but particularly folic acid, may contribute to reducing homocysteine so do not worry if your multivitamin does not contain all three.

e. CALCIUM SUPPLEMENTATION may be required if you avoid dairy produce due to lactose intolerance or adopt a vegan lifestyle. For normal people, more than 70% of calcium is taken up from dairy produce although fortified foods such as bread and some cereals are also important sources. All flour in the UK is fortified with calcium except wholemeal which naturally contains 380mg calcium per kilogram. As a rough guide, you need 800-1500 mg of calcium per day and 3 cups of milk (or yoghurt) will provide about 900 mg. See Table 3 in Chapter 1 for other food sources of calcium. Calcium supplements are one of the most popular mineral supplements in the USA and UK.

Again, it is for you to judge whether you have enough dairy produce and/or fortified food each day to obtain the necessary 800-1500 mg of calcium. Special groups of people who are more likely to require calcium supplements are young children (800 mg) to ensure they have strong bones as well as pregnant and nursing mothers (1200-1500 mg), menopausal women and elderly people (1500 mg). See details for some of these groups below and consult with your doctor about supplementation.

If you do decide to take a calcium supplement then be aware that calcium may inhibit the absorption of iron. Check to make sure that your multivitamin does not contain both iron and calcium. In addition, fibre in food may bind to calcium and inhibit uptake so vegans/vegetarians beware. It is therefore recommended that calcium pills are taken 1-2 hr after a meal and no more than 500 mg should be taken each time. Make sure that you have sufficient vitamin D (see above) which will aid in the absorption of calcium.

f. GLUCOSAMINE is taken by people from middle age onwards for the reduction of joint pain and inflammation, often associated with osteoarthritis, and to assist with joint mobility. Over 2 million people in the UK suffer from osteoarthritis with the average age of onset about 45 years old. The dose usually recommended orally is 1500 mg per day and should be taken for 6-8 weeks to see if symptoms improve. Glucosamine is not a registered medicine in the UK and therefore is a supplement which may or may not provide relief. Generally, glucosamine is safe to take long-term except for people with allergies to shellfish. Sometimes glucosamine is taken with chondroitin sulphate as this combination may provide further benefit for people with osteoarthritis (see reference 108). A recent study concluded, however, that glucosamine sulphate (1500 mg daily) was ineffective for treating hip osteoarthritis (see reference 109). A controversy thus exists so the best thing to do is to try glucosamine if you suffer from osteoarthritis and see if your symptoms improve. Also, note the warning in Table 3, Chapter 1, about not taking glucosamine **sulphate** but glucosamine **hydrochloride** instead, if you have high blood pressure.

SUMMARY RECOMMENDATION FOR "NORMAL" HEALTHY PEOPLE 19-59 YEARS OLD

+++ vitamin D

BUT if you do not eat at least 5 fruit or vegetable portions per day (over 80% of this group) and also do not have sufficient dairy produce in

your diet then you may require supplementation with one or more of the following:

+++ multivitamin (preferably without vitamin A)

+++ vitamin D and calcium

++ omega-3 fish oil (not cod liver oil)

++ glucosamine for osteoarthritis sufferers usually over 40 years old

++ vitamin B from multivitamin (see above) or from a separate supplement to get higher levels of B-6 and B-12

All daily

NB: If you are taking any medicines then check with your medical advisor that these will not interact with the vitamin pills.

ii. PREGNANT WOMEN Women intending to conceive or who are pregnant are recommended to take 400 micrograms of **folic acid (vitamin B9)** per day as a supplement to reduce the chances of spina bifida. If a spina bifida baby was born previously, this should be increased to 5mg of folic acid. More recently, the Department of Health has also advised pregnant and breast-feeding women to take a 10 microgram per day **vitamin D** supplement to avoid problems with skeletal development (rickets). This is especially important in the winter when vitamin D cannot be made by the body due to lack of exposure to the sun. Iron supplements are not recommended by the UK Food Standards Agency unless the woman is anaemic. Pregnant women should be tested for anaemia routinely. Many women take a multivitamin-mineral supplement prior to and during pregnancy. This is beneficial for those foolish enough to smoke and drink whilst pregnant but **make sure that such multivitamins do not contain vitamin A which can cause foetal malformations.** Many multivitamins carry no warning over the dangers of vitamin A to the baby. Avoid foods and supplements like liver, pate and fish oils (eg. cod liver oil) with high levels of vitamin A (**http://www.eatwell.gov.uk**). Maternal omega-3 fish oil supplementation during pregnancy has also been shown to be safe for the foetus and infant, and may have beneficial effects on the child's eye and hand coordination, although more evidence is required before strong recommendation can be made. Tinned or fresh mackerel, salmon, trout, herring, kippers, pilchards, anchovies, fresh tuna (no more than one 6 oz tuna steak per week) and sardines naturally contain beneficial omega-3 oils. Avoid eating shark, swordfish and marlin steaks which can be high in mercury (see reference 97).

SUMMARY RECOMMENDATION

+++ folic acid

+++ vitamin D (usually D3 recommended)

++ omega-3 fish oils, 1000 mg per day, if intolerant of 2-4 portions of oily fish each week

All daily

iii. BREAST FEEDING WOMEN like pregnant women should boost their intake of **vitamin D.** In addition, if the pregnant or nursing mother does not have a diet high in calcium, since she may avoid dairy products through allergy etc, then a **calcium supplement** may be required and she should consult with her GP. Multivitamins may be recommended, but those made especially for nursing mothers should be used.

SUMMARY RECOMMENDATION

+++   vitamin D

++   multivitamin

+   calcium

All daily

iv. BABIES AND INFANTS less than 6 months old and fed on breast milk or formula milk should not need supplements. If breast-fed then after 6 months **vitamin A, C and D supplements** (as liquid drops) may be required but only under direction of a health visitor/doctor. These can be continued until 5 yr old if the child eats poorly or is not exposed to the sun for short times.

SUMMARY RECOMMENDATION

+   vitamins A, C and D (liquid drops)

All daily

v. SCHOOL CHILDREN may have poor diets with less than half surveyed eating the 5 a day fruit and vegetables required. Approximately, 20% of 4-18 year olds eat no fruit at all (see reference 110). In addition, about 20% of UK teenagers are obese with numbers having tripled since 1980. Up to 10% of teenage girls may also be vegetarians or on special diets. It is no wonder that teenagers are reported to have low intakes of vitamin A, D and riboflavin (vitamin B2) as well as the minerals, calcium, zinc, iron and magnesium. Lectures on healthy eating are often ignored. It has been shown that **taking a multivitamin supplement** is highly beneficial for teens and associated with healthier lifestyles (see reference 111). Since over 70% of teenage girls may also be vitamin D deficient (see reference 112), supplementation may be highly beneficial. Multivitamins for teens contain 2.5-5 micrograms (100-200 IU) of vitamin D.

SUMMARY RECOMMENDATION

+++ multivitamin

++   vitamin D daily but only if multivitamin not taken daily

vi. WOMEN WITH HEAVY PERIODS are particularly prone to **iron deficiency anaemia** due to excessive loss of blood and will benefit from iron supplementation under supervision. Teenage girls with diets rich in sugar, snacks and crisps, which interfere with iron uptake, may also be in need of additional iron. Eating vitamin C–rich foods such as fruit, juices and vegetables (see Table 2, Chapter 1) will aid in iron absorption. Women using oral contraceptives may have reduced bleeding during periods and are less likely to require iron supplements. Vitamin D is recommended (400 IU =10 micrograms daily) during the winter months or if not exposed to sunlight for about 15 min twice per week without sunscreen greater than factor 8.

SUMMARY RECOMMENDATION

++   iron

++   vitamin D

Both daily

vii. MENOPAUSAL AND POST-MENOPAUSAL WOMEN

Recommending supplements for these groups of women is controversial. Neither the Foods Standards Agency nor the British Nutrition Foundation recommends specific supplementation for women at these stages, although they emphasise the importance of a balanced diet. Women on iron supplements can stop using these when menstrual bleeding reduces during the menopause. For women not on Hormone Replacement Therapy (HRT), a whole range of supplements have been recommended to alleviate menopausal symptoms and bone loss resulting from osteoporosis or bone thinning and resulting in increased fractures. These supplements include vitamins A, B, C, D, E and K, as well as the minerals, calcium and magnesium, and plant/herb extracts containing phytoestrogens such as dong quai, black cohosh, red clover and soya. Evidence is limited or controversial as to the beneficial effects of using most of these. The case, however, for the use of calcium and vitamin D supplements is gradually being accepted as is the need for a revision upwards of the safe upper limits in the use of vitamin D (see reference 113). Old upper safety limits for vitamin D were originally set over 30 years ago to prevent rickets. **Evidence now indicates that supplementation with 700-800 IU (17.5-20 microgram) vitamin D results in fewer fractures, with or without a**

calcium supplement. Cod liver oil contains not only high levels of vitamin D but also vitamin A which can be toxic so it is better to use a pure vitamin D supplement. Vitamin E and black cohosh may also reduce hot flushes, but beware of using any herbs with the Pill or HRT.

SUMMARY RECOMMENDATION

+++   vitamin D

+   calcium

Both daily

viii. PEOPLE OVER 50-60 YR OLD   must avoid at all costs:

"THE DOWNWARD SPIRAL OF AGING"

This process results from older people:

1.   Eating less or buying lower quality food because of reduced incomes

2.   Eating less food due to dental problems and inability to chew effectively

3.   Having a reduced efficiency for digestion and absorption of food by the gut which may be related to loss of acid production in the stomach

4.   Living alone due to loss of partner or divorce and a reduced incentive to prepare regular and well balanced meals

5.   Confined indoors, away from sunlight, due to illness or social isolation, resulting in vitamin deficiency

6.   Commonly taking medications such as antibiotics that may interfere with vitamin and mineral absorption

7.   Suffering malnutrition as a result of 1-6 (above) and losing weight, strength and energy for exercise

8.   Having little exercise which accelerates loss of muscle and bone mass (see, "Sarcopenia" and "Osteoporosis" in Chapter 11 of IYL, pages 217-220), reduced strength and results in frailty, more frequent falls, fractures and infections

9.   Loss of independence

10. Admission into Care Home or Hospital

Figure 3. Showing components of the "Downward Spiral of Aging"

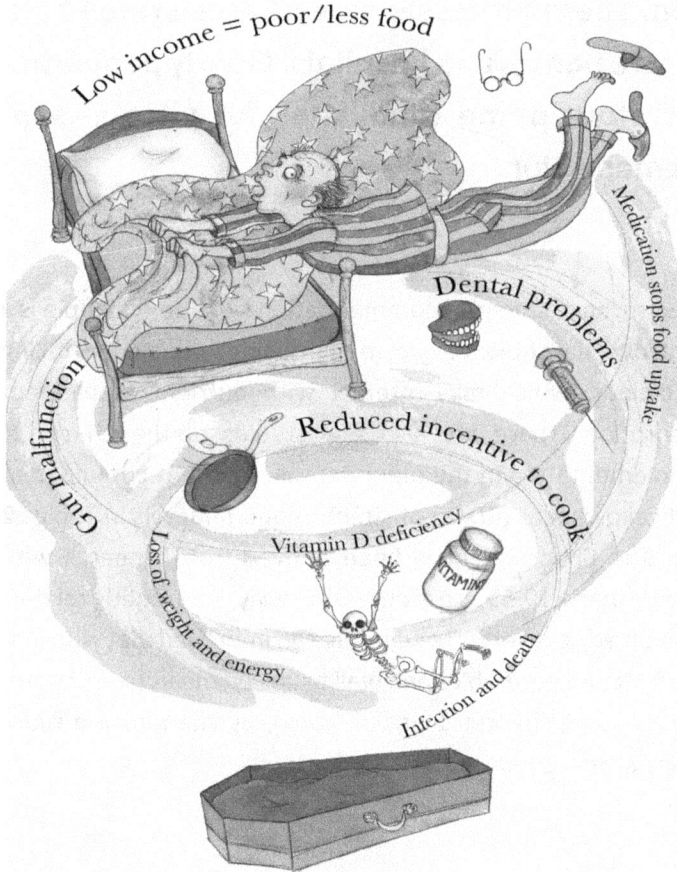

Low income = poor/less food

Medication stops food uptake

Dental problems

Gut malfunction

Reduced incentive to cook

Vitamin D deficiency

Loss of weight and energy

Infection and death

VITAMIN

The aging process is thus accelerated by a downward spiral of malnutrition, weakness, frailty, reduced immune efficiency and infection. These processes may be accelerated both in care homes and hospitals. Elderly people are therefore prime candidates for vitamin supplementation.

Even so, supplement recommendation for elderly people is a controversial subject since so many older people are taking medicines, which may interact with nutrient/supplement absorption. There are also few studies of the effects of supplementation in the older person. All the recommended daily allowances (RDAs) of vitamins and minerals in Tables 2 and 3 in Chapter 1 have been derived from research with people in the 19-59 age group. Obviously, if an elderly relative is involved, it is better to supervise an improved diet with 5-a-day fruit and vegetables and well balanced meals (see Chapter 1 of IYL and Chapter 1 of this book), as vitamins are more easily absorbed naturally from food.

A **multivitamin supplement** seems the obvious choice and yet some trials of the beneficial effects of multivitamin supplements have failed to detect any reduction in infection rates in elderly people over 65 yr old (see reference 114). Possibly, these negative results occurred because some of the vitamins and minerals in the multivitamin pills interfered with the absorption of each other. Also, these trials tended to **use healthy, older people living at home** rather than more **nutritionally-deprived people in care homes and hospitals**. Indeed, a few trials with multivitamins have recorded reduced infection rates in institutionalized older people (see reference 115). Perhaps these contrary results confirm that providing people have adequate diets then at any age vitamin supplementation has only limited benefits.

Trials with individual vitamins, however, have achieved more promising results. Thus, the case can now be made for the use of **vitamin B and D supplements in older people** but only after the health professional confirms that these do not interfere with any medication taken.

A deficiency of B vitamins may not only impair memory and alertness but can also result in reduced energy for exercise as well as anaemia. There are also indications that B vitamins can protect against strokes, heart problems and Alzheimer's disease. **Vitamin B12 deficiency** occurs in 10-15% of 60+ year olds and can result in anaemia and dementia-like symptoms which can be treated either by monthly injections of 1 mg or by supplements of 100-200 micrograms per day, depending on the extent of deficiency. Recently, **vitamin B9 (folic acid) supplements of 800 micrograms per day** have also been shown to improve the memories and brain power of 50 to 70 year olds (see reference 116). There is also discussion about the **role of vitamin B6** in dementia and mental processes. **On balance, vitamin B supplementation would seem worthwhile in elderly people assuming no interaction with any drugs prescribed.** In the USA, there has been fortification of cereals with folic acid for the last 10 years.

There is some controversy regarding **supplementation with Vitamin D** but in people, such as the elderly deprived of sunlight, **a dose of 700-800 IU (17.5-20 micrograms) per day** is recommended to reduce falls and fractures (see, previous section, "menopausal and post-menopausal women"). The use of vitamin D supplements may also increase life expectancy significantly (see reference 117). In addition, since vitamin D and calcium work together in the body, it is recommended

to take a calcium supplement of not more than 1500 mg per day to slow down bone loss in the elderly. Again, controversy exists over the use of these supplements so consult your doctor first.

Studies have also discussed the **benefits of taking vitamins C and E as well as selenium and zinc**. Again, there is controversy since there are reports that using C, E and selenium might increase the incidence of certain cancers. In contrast, there is evidence for a protective role with vitamins C and E against Alzheimer's disease but only at much higher doses than present in multivitamins. Thus, 500 mg of vitamin C and 400 IU vitamin E would be required and there is evidence that vitamin E at this level could be harmful. Thus, improving the diet rather than overdosing on vitamins C and E would be optimal. Selenium is an important antioxidant, levels of which have been declining in the UK diet with the institutionalised elderly at the greatest risk of deficiency. A **supplement of 50 micrograms per day** can be taken with no side effects but it is better to confirm deficiency with a blood test first. The case for **supplementing with zinc (10mg per day) is strongest** for elderly people to boost their immune system and prevent infections such as pneumonia.

Many elderly people also take **fish oil capsules regularly (1000 mg per day)** to maintain and improve joint flexibility and relieve arthritic pain. In addition, fish oils may have many other benefits such as reducing the risk of heart disease, strokes and cancer. Again, unfortunately, scientific opinion differs as to the benefits of taking fish oils although the weight of evidence does seem favorable. In addition, recent research has also shown that omega-3 fish oils can help combat Alzheimer's disease but only in certain people **without a gene predisposing them to developing Alzheimer's** (see reference 118). Taking omega-3 fish oils, which are present naturally in sardines, mackerel, herrings and salmon, is harmless and is therefore recommended. Do buy a good quality omega-3 free of dioxin and mercury.

The Food Standards Agency (www.**eatwell.gov.uk**) recommends that elderly people avoid fish liver oils, such as **COD LIVER OIL** supplements, as they contain high quantities of vitamin A which can result in loss of bone density, osteoporosis and increase in

> bone fractures. Cod liver oil supplements for elderly people have recently been recommended by a TV doctor who should know better.

Finally, many elderly people also take **glucosamine sulphate** supplements for osteoarthritis which affects the joints. This supplement may reduce joint pain and inflammation and assist with joint mobility. The dose usually recommended orally is 1500 mg per day and it should be taken for 6-8 weeks to see if symptoms improve. Glucosamine is not a registered medicine in the UK and therefore is a supplement which may or may not provide relief. Generally, glucosamine is safe to take long-term except for people with allergies to shellfish. Sometimes glucosamine is taken with chondroitin sulphate as this combination may provide further benefit for people with osteoarthritis (see reference 108). A recent study (see reference 109) concluded, however, that glucosamine sulphate (1500 mg daily) was ineffective for treating hip osteoarthritis. A controversy thus exists so that the best thing to do is to try glucosamine if you suffer from osteoarthritis and see if your symptoms improve. Check Table 3, Chapter 1, for use of glucosamine hydrochloride instead of sulphate in cases of high blood pressure.

SUMMARY RECOMMENDATION

NB: If you are taking any medicines then check with your medical advisor that these will not interact with the vitamin pills.

+++ multivitamin for elderly in care/hospital (preferably without vitamin A)

+++ vitamin D* and calcium**

++ omega-3 fish oil (not cod liver oil)

++ glucosamine for osteoarthritis sufferers

++ vitamin B* from multivitamin (above) but if very deficient in vitamin B 12 then 1 mg per month of B 12 injected or a 100-200 microgram tablet daily dissolved under the tongue

All the above daily

*NB: Both vitamins B and D may be present in the multivitamin (as in the Boots multivitamin for the over 50s) in which case these may not have to be taken again separately. If levels of vitamins B and D are very low in the multivitamin, it may be necessary to take these separately. If the multivitamin contains iron, this may compete with calcium for absorption by the gut, in which case take your calcium supplement (with food but not with caffeine drinks) some hours after the multivitamin.

**There is some discussion as to whether calcium supplements can cause hardening of the arteries and heart attacks/strokes but further research is needed. In the meantime, if over 70 yr old, eat more high calcium-rich foods and reduce calcium supplements (for reassurance see reference 119). This study looked at over 36,000, 50-79 yr old women and found no adverse effects of calcium supplements.

ix. PEOPLE IN HOSPITAL/CARE HOMES. These include sick people with long stays in hospital and disabled or others, such as Alzheimer's patients, in care. This group includes elderly people (see above) who are likely to be malnourished and would benefit from a multivitamin and, if confined indoors, also vitamin D. To avoid interactions with any medication, check with a health professional before taking supplements.

SUMMARY RECOMMENDATION

+++ multivitamin (without vitamin A if possible)

+++ vitamin D

Both daily

x. CIGARETTE SMOKERS are damaging the DNA and organs throughout their bodies, including the lungs, gut and heart, due to the oxidative stress resulting from the chemicals in cigarette smoke. This will often lead to cancer, cardiovascular disease and accelerated aging. Smoking reduces levels of antioxidants such as vitamins C and E which can defend the body against the ravages of smoking (see reference 120). In addition, it has been shown that levels of the B vitamins, such as B6, B9 and B12, are also lower in smokers.

RECENT RESEARCH HAS SHOWN THAT SMOKING INCREASES

THE RISK OF DEMENTIA AND ALZHEIMER'S DISEASE

A vitamin C supplement of 1000 mg per day has been reported to significantly reduce the loss of vitamin E caused by smoking. It is also better to take a separate vitamin B supplement since multivitamins often contain vitamin A.

DO NOT TAKE VITAMIN A OR VITAMIN E SUPPLEMENTS IF YOU SMOKE AS THESE MAY INCREASE THE INCIDENCE OF LUNG CANCER.

SUMMARY RECOMMENDATION

+++ vitamin C

++ vitamin B

++ vitamin D

All daily

xi. DRINKERS are likely to be to be suffering from multiple vitamin deficiencies. This is true not only for alcoholics but also for binge drinkers at the weekend and for people drinking regularly throughout the week with friends or during work. This vitamin deficiency results from both a poor diet, which drinkers often have, and from alcohol inhibiting the uptake of vitamins and increasing their breakdown in the stomach. **Vitamins particularly affected are B1 (thiamine), B2 (riboflavin), B6 (pyridoxine), B9 (folic acid) and vitamin C.** The extent of any deficiency will depend upon the amount and regularity of drInking as well as upon the normal intake of vitamins in the diet. In addition, vitamins A, D and E as well as vital minerals such as calcium, zinc, iron and magnesium may also be deficient in alcoholics. The results of these alcohol-induced deficiencies will vary from one person to another but can have serious consequences. Thus, folic acid deficiency has been reported to be linked to anaemia, cancer of the colon, Alzheimer's and foetal damage, while **long-term thiamine (B1) deficiency can result in severe brain damage and dementia.**

RECENT WORK HAS SHOWN THAT WHEN HEAVY DRINKING IS ASSOCIATED WITH SMOKING THEN THE AGE OF ONSET OF ALZHEIMER'S DISEASE CAN BE 6-7 YEARS EARLIER
(see reference 121)

The research showed:

- Heavy drinkers developed Alzheimer's 4.8 years earlier than non-drinkers or light drinkers.

- Heavy smokers developed Alzheimer's 2.3 years earlier than non-smokers or light smokers.

- Those people who drank and smoked heavily but also had the APOE4 gene, which increases the risk of

Alzheimer's, developed the disease 8.5 years earlier than those without the three risk factors.

HEAVY DRINKERS WERE DEFINED AS THOSE WHO HAD MORE THAN TWO DRINKS EVERY DAY, WHILE HEAVY SMOKERS HAD 20 OR MORE CIGARETTES PER DAY.

A TRUE AND SAD STORY

This involved my sister who died recently from Alzheimer's disease at the age of 66. She was an ex beauty queen, London fashion model and then a famous astrologer. She wrote for many of the daily and weekend national newspapers, including the Sunday Mirror, Daily Express and Daily Star, as well as appearing regularly on Living TV. Unfortunately, her astrology writing meant that for many years she was confined for months on end in her study trying to meet deadlines for her 12 monthly astrology guides published each year. In addition, like many people, she had marital problems, and the stress of these and her need to meet tight deadlines resulted in more and more excessive smoking and drinking. Eventually, I noticed changes in her appearance and eyesight both of which gradually degenerated. Like the rest of her family, however, I had no idea as to the level of her drinking until large numbers of empty vodka bottles were found in her study. Her behaviour became more and more eccentric and her short-term memory practically non-existent. Eventually her appearance, memory and behaviour necessitated medical scrutiny and resulted in the diagnosis of Alzheimer's disease. This was followed by her institutionalization and, finally, her death in just a few years. Her decline was no doubt hastened by a poor diet, including excessive amounts of cheese, which would have raised her cholesterol levels to possibly contribute to her early onset of dementia. Thus, I lost a beautiful and dearly beloved sister to excessive stress, drinking and smoking coupled to a poor diet – factors that often go hand-in-hand.

DOES ANY OF THIS SOUND FAMILIAR TO YOU?

SUMMARY RECOMMENDATION

It is difficult to be precise in making recommendations for drinkers as a lot will depend upon the amount drunk and how frequently. Alcoholics may need emergency treatment and institutionalizing with daily injection of high dose vitamins. Regular and binge drinkers would do well to take:

+++   a multivitamin tablet daily

+++   vitamin B complex 100-300 mg daily, the dose taken depending upon both the amount drunk daily and the nutritional value of the diet

+++   vitamin C by eating more fruit but also by at least a 500 mg tablet daily

xii. DIABETICS There are about 2 million diagnosed diabetic adults in England, with numbers rising at an alarming rate. With a body mass index (BMI) in excess of 30 there is as much as a ten-fold increase in risk of becoming diabetic. There are also ethnic groups at particular risk of developing diabetes including Afro-Caribbeans and Asians. **Most importantly, recent research indicates that levels of specific vitamins can be linked to both the risk of developing diabetes as well as preventing the complications resulting in heart disease, strokes, blindness, kidney and nerve damage.** Thus, **low levels of vitamin D**, due to low intake or lack of exposure to the sun, may increase the risk of developing diabetes. This might explain why dark-skinned people, who are less able to make their own vitamin D, are more prone to develop diabetes. In addition, low vitamin D levels in diabetics are correlated with complications such as cardiovascular disease (see review reference 122). Even more recently, research has shown that **diabetics have blood levels of vitamin B1 (thiamine) which are about 75% lower than in normal people**. Since thiamine is important in maintaining healthy blood vessels then this thiamine deficiency in diabetics may be linked to the many complications of diabetes (see reference 123).

SUMMARY RECOMMENDATION

+++ vitamin D, some people have a 33% reduced risk of diabetes if taking 800 IU (20 micrograms) vitamin D together with 1200 mg of calcium daily. Consult your doctor

+++ vitamin B1 (thiamine), supplementa tion of diabetic patients' diet with thiamine is on trial, but it is worth while taking a vitamin B supplement in a multivitamin until optimal levels have been determined

Both daily

xiii. PEOPLE WITH GUT PROBLEMS There are a range of conditions that can lead to the poor absorption (malabsorption) of nutrients, such as vitamins and minerals, from food. Thus, malabsorption can occur with **Crohn's disease, ulcerative colitis, inflammatory bowel syndrome, coeliac disease, food allergy/intolerance, gut infections and cancer**. Such diseases will have to be diagnosed and treated medically. In some of these conditions, vitamin supplementation is unnecessary as with allergic or intolerance reactions to food, for example, **coeliac disease** caused by sensitivity to the gluten protein present in cereals or with **lactose intolerance** to dairy products. Simply avoiding these foods may rectify the problem. With other conditions, including **Crohn's disease**, multiple vitamin and mineral deficiencies can occur. Thus, deficiencies in many vitamins including A, B1, B2, B6, folic acid, B12, E and K as well as the minerals, zinc, calcium and magnesium have been found (reviewed in reference 124). Likewise with **cancer of the gut, pancreas, liver or gallbladder,** there may be multiple impairment of the digestion and absorption of vitamins and minerals and other nutrients. Whether supplements are required and how to take them will depend upon **diagnosis of the type and severity of the disease**. In some cases, adjustments to the diet will be sufficient (eg. coeliac disease) while in others, supplements will need to be injected or given directly into the veins (cancer).

SUMMARY RECOMMENDATION

+++   multivitamin daily BUT depends on which disease and it's severity.

Supplementation should be given under the direction of a health professional.

xiv. OVERWEIGHT OR OBESE PEOPLE In the UK more than 50% of adults are overweight (BMI 25-30) and about 23% of these are obese (BMI over 30). Many overweight people have poor diets rich in fatty and sugary foods and alcohol but low in fruit, vegetables and dairy products. In addition, they may struggle unsuccessfully with various diets such as the Atkins which are low in fruits and vegetables. The end result is that overweight people often have vitamin and mineral deficiencies but particularly vitamins B6 (pyridoxine), C, D and E, and if they are dieting they may lack minerals such as iron, calcium and zinc. Taking a multivitamin and mineral supplement is recommended regardless of whether dieting or not. Vitamin D deficiency has now been shown to be higher in obese people than in the normal population (see reference 125).

SUMMARY RECOMMENDATION

+++   a multivitamin tablet

+++   vitamin D (10 micrograms, 400IU)

Both daily

xv. VEGANS, VEGETARIANS AND PEOPLE ON

DIETS are likely to be deficient in certain key vitamins and minerals. This group will include not only overweight people (see: "Overweight or Obese People", above) but also those on special diets such as vegans and vegetarians. Between 3% and 7% of the UK population are vegetarians and these include vegans who avoid all food of animal origin. Sometimes, people adopting a vegetarian lifestyle may have mineral or vitamin deficiencies due to a lack of knowledge of the optimal foods to eat. Vegetarians may need supplements containing vitamins B12 and D as well as calcium, iron and zinc, all of which are present in meat and dairy produce. **Vitamin B12 is a particular need in vegetarians** since it is not present in plant tissues and deficiency may lead to anaemia and nerve damage. Yeast extracts and Marmite are sources of B12 as are some foods such as soya milk and breakfast cereals fortified with this vitamin (read the labels). **Vitamin D deficiency is widespread in the normal UK population but some vegetarians (especially vegans) will be even more deficient** since dietary sources of vitamin D are of animal origin, including liver, dairy produce and oily fish. Some dairy-free milks and margarines are fortified with vitamin D (but with very low levels) and free of harmful hydrogenated fats (trans fats). **Calcium, iron and zinc can all be obtained from the vegeta-**

rian diet. Details of plant sources of these minerals are given in Table 3 of Chapter 1.

SUMMARY RECOMMENDATION

+++   a multivitamin tablet for dieters

+++   vitamin B12 for vegetarians with 100-200* microgram tablet dissolved under the tongue

+++   vitamin D (10 micrograms, 400IU)

All daily

* there is disagreement as to the exact dose of vitamin B12 required as a supplement.

xvi. PEOPLE WHO EXERCISE REGULARLY should not normally require any further vitamin and mineral supplementation in addition to those recommended for "Normal Healthy People 19-59 Years Old" (see page 74, above). During exercise, the body uses more oxygen which results in the formation of additional oxygen radicals that may damage the tissues. Research, however, seems to indicate that the body can compensate naturally for this additional oxidative stress by increased production of antioxidant enzymes without the need to take antioxidant supplements (see review reference 126). It is, however, important to emphasise that people taking regular exercise need to have a balanced diet to provide the necessary calories for energy production, protein for tissue repair and fruit and vegetables as sources of antioxidants. **With endurance athletes, such as regular marathon runners, tri-athletes, cyclists etc, there is, however, some evidence that antioxidant supplements may offer protection** against the very high levels (10-20 times resting state levels) of radicals generated by these sports. Thus, an **increased intake of vitamin E may be protective** but precise levels are unknown although 100-200 IU per day has been recommended. In addition, since some athletes may restrict their intake of calories and certain food groups, they may have vitamin or mineral deficiencies. A **multivitamin-mineral supplement containing a range of B-vitamins** will ensure that energy production and muscle repair are optimal.

SUMMARY RECOMMENDATION

++   vitamin E may protect **endurance athletes** against oxidative stress

++   a multivitamin-mineral supplement for **endurance athletes** will ensure that performance is not inhibited by deficiencies

Both daily

FROM THE ABOVE, WE CAN ESTIMATE THAT ABOUT 45 MILLION PEOPLE FROM A POPULATION IN THE UK OF 61.4 MILLION BELONG TO GROUPS LIKELY TO BENEFIT FROM VITAMIN/MINERAL SUPPLEMENTS

TIPS ON BUYING VITAMINS AND MINERALS Deciding which make of vitamins/minerals to buy can be a difficult task with prices for apparently similar products being highly variable. In addition, supplements can be expensive and nobody wishes to spend more than necessary. Having decided, from reading the above and Chapter 1, the type and strength of vitamins required then it is essential to be confident that the brand(s) chosen meets your requirements. Remember, the following points only need to be considered before your **first** purchase:

1. Read the labels on the bottle and check that the pills contain the appropriate vitamin/mineral dose required and are not out of date.

2. Also look for any **warnings of interactions with certain medicines given in the instructions in each packet** (see below, page 142).

3. When buying multivitamins, make sure that you purchase **the correct type** required i.e. for children, pregnant or nursing mothers, or people over 50 yr old etc.

4. With a multivitamin, double check that the RDA (recommended daily allowance) for vitamin A or beta-carotene **is not above 100%.**

5. Many vitamins are synthetic rather than "natural" or "organic" and there is "evidence" that **some natural vitamins**, such as vitamin E, are not only **absorbed more effectively in the gut but utilised better** by the body. Natural vitamin E will be labelled "d-alpha-tocopherol" and synthetic "dl-alpha-tocopherol".

6. **There is very little regulation regarding the production of supplements** and no guarantee that they contain the amount of

vitamin/mineral written on the label. If you really need to check the quality of supplements then enquire in the shop and failing a satisfactory answer (probably) ask for a contact telephone number. A reputable manufacturer should be able to provide answers/proof of their quality control processes. In the UK, information about vitamins and supplements is available in Holland and Barrett and Boots stores from trained personnel who should help. In the USA, supplements can be checked out at:

www.supplementquality.com/testing/Quality_seals.html

Note that the European Commission has a Working Group considering setting maximum and minimum levels of vitamins and minerals in foodstuffs such as supplements (see reference 127).

FOR FUN WITH THE CHILDREN why not carry out a simple experiment. Vitamin and mineral pills not only contain the supplement required but also fillers, binders and coatings to stabilise and hold the pill together. **It is worthwhile**

checking if the pills taken dissolve in the gut to release their contents for absorption by the body or whether they pass straight through the gut into the toilet. Simply place some vinegar in a heat-proof container and heat on a hotplate to 98° F = body temperature (take care with the hotplate). Put the test pill in the container, maintain the temperature and stir every few minutes without touching the pill. The pill should dissolve by 30-45 min unless it is labelled "enteric coated" or "slow release" which should be resistant to the acid in the stomach represented by the vinegar. If it dissolves too quickly then this is also of concern as the contents may be broken down and destroyed in the stomach.

TIPS ON TAKING VITAMIN/MINERAL SUPPLEMENTS

1. **To aid in their absorption, these should generally be taken with a meal or snack**. This is especially important with the fat-soluble vitamins such as vitamins A, D

and E, beta carotene and coenzyme Q10. Make sure that the **food contains a little fat** (no, not a bacon buttie!) which will aid in the absorption of these latter vitamins. Excess of these fat-soluble vitamins are stored in the body and therefore do not exceed the correct dose.

2. **Other vitamins, such as B and C, dissolve in water** and will rapidly pass out of the body in the urine unless taken with food. Some vitamins, such as vitamin C, are sold as "enteric-coated" or "slow release" and will survive passage through the acid in the stomach into the small intestine for better absorption.

3. **Do not take your vitamins with hot drinks or drinks containing caffeine** which is present in tea, coffee, colas etc. Caffeine inhibits the absorption of some vitamins and minerals, such as iron, and

stimulates the loss of others, such as calcium, from the body.

4. **Calcium may inhibit the absorption of iron** so do not take both at the same time. In addition, **fibre in food may bind to calcium** and inhibit uptake so vegans/vegetarians beware. Therefore, **take calcium pills 1-2 hr after a meal** and no more than 500mg should be taken each time.

5. Most people take vitamins as tablets or capsules, however, **there are liquid vitamins** for people who find pills difficult to swallow. Liquid vitamins tend to be expensive and could potentially lose more of their activity in the acid of the stomach than tablet forms, especially more than enteric-coated pills.

INTERACTIONS OF VITAMINS WITH MEDICINES

IF YOU HAVE A MEDICAL CONDITION IT IS MOST IMPORTANT TO CONSULT YOUR DOCTOR BEFORE TAKING SUPPLEMENTS.

It is natural for sick people to take supplements in the hope of "strengthening" their immune systems and speeding recovery. Cancer patients, in particular, are amongst the highest users of supplements. There are **many accounts of the interactions of vitamins and minerals with medicines** with some of these scientifically proven while others are more theoretical and the basis of cautionary advice. For example:

1. There is much cautionary advice about cancer patients not taking high doses of antioxidants like vitamins A and E as these may not only interfere

with the action of chemotherapeutic drugs but also stimulate cancer cell growth.

2. Folic acid (vitamin B-9) can interfere with some drugs used to treat epilepsy and inflammation.

3. Riboflavin (vitamin B-3) impairs the activity of some (streptomycin, erythromycin and tetracyclines) but not all (chloramphenicol, penicillin) antibiotics.

4. Pyrodoxine (vitamin B-6) supplements reduce the effects of the drug, levodopa, used for treating Parkinson's disease.

5. Vitamin E taken with the blood thinning drug, warfarin, increases the risk of abnormal bleeding. Vitamin E also reduces the body's uptake of the antidepressant, desimpramine.

6. Calcium (carbonate) may interact with Levothyroxine, a drug used to treat thyroid disease and cancer.

In addition, some drugs will affect vitamins and minerals in the body. For example:

1. The cytotoxic antifungal agents, actinomycin and imidazole, may interfere with vitamin D activity.

2. Metaformin is used for treating diabetes and increases the risk of vitamin B-12 deficiency.

The next book in the series is:

It's Your Life – Exercise For All Ages

For the complete guide to a healthy life:

*It's Your Life: End the confusion from
inconsistent health advice*

Reference sources for conclusions

Chapter 1

76. **www.prnewswire.co.uk/cgi/news/release?id=96968**

77. British Association of Parental and Enteral Nutrition (BAPEN) report, 2005, **www.bapen.org.uk**

78. Joanne Blythman, "The Food We Eat" (Michael Joseph 1996).

79. Joanne Blythman, "Bad Food Britain: How A Nation Ruined Its Appetite" (Fourth Estate 2006).

80. **www.food.gov.uk/foodindustry/famingfood/organicfood**

81. Organic Food: Facts and Figures, 2006, **www.soilassociation.org**

82. **www.food.gov.uk/news/newsarchive/2009**

83. Dangour and colleagues, American Journal Clinical Nutrition, Vol. 90, pages 680-685, 2009.

84. Mozaffarian and colleagues, Journal American Medical Assoc., Vol. 289, pages 1659-1666, 2003.

85. "Irradiated Food in Europe and the UK", The Food Commission, July 2002:

   www.foodcomm.org.uk/irradiation_probs.htm

86. Giannakourou and Taoukis, Food Chemistry, Vol. 83, pages 33-41, 2003.

87. Vallejo and colleagues, Journal of the Science of Food and Agriculture, Vol. 83, pages 1511-1516, 2003.

88. **http://ods.od.nih.gov**

89. **lpi.oregonstate.edu/infocenter**

90. **www.food.gov.uk/multimedia/webpage/vitandmin/** Then open up pdf entitled "Safe upper limits for vitamins and minerals, 2003".

91. Jenkins and colleagues, Canadian Medical Association Journal fact sheet, 2008, see:

   www.cmaj.ca/cgi/content/full/178/2/150

Chapter 2

92. www.netdoctor.co.uk/dietandnutriton/feature/vitamins

93. www.food.gov.uk/science/dietarysurveys/ndnsdocuments

94. www.5aday.nhs.uk Open up "The school fruit and vegetable scheme".

95. Hypponen and Power, Journal Clinical Nutrition, Vol. 85, pages 860-868, 2007.

96. Lavie and colleagues, Journal American College of Cardiology, Vol. 54, pages 585-594, 2009.

97. www.food.gov.uk/science/surveillance/fsis2003/fsis402003

98. Ann Intern Med. 2006;145:364-371.

99. www.ajcn.org/cgi/reprint/85/1/265S.pdf?ck=nck

100. Stidley, Cancer Research, Vol.70, pages 568-574, 2010.

101. http://www.food.gov.uk/multimedia/pdfs/vitmin2003.pdf

102. Pauling L. "How to Live Longer and Feel Better", New York: WH Freeman, 1986.

103. Orr and Sohal, Science, Vol. 263, pages 1128-1130, 1994.

104. news.bbc.co.uk/2/hi/health/4520727

105. http://www.thecochranelibrary.com, 2009, issue 1, Nikolova and colleagues.

106. Tucker, American Journal Clinical Nutrition, Vol. 71, pages 514-522, 2000.

107. Wald and colleagues, British Medical Journal, Vol. 333, pages 1114-1117.

108. Tat and colleagues, Arthritis Research Therapy, 9, R117, 2007.

109. Bijlsma and Lafeber, Annals Internal Medicine, Vol. 148, pages 315-316, 2008.

110. www.nutrition.org.uk/home

111. Reaves and colleagues, J. American Dietetic Association, Vol. 106, pages 2018-2023, 2006.

112. Das and colleagues, Archives Disease in Childhood, Vol. 91, pages 569-572, 2006.

113 Vieth, editorial in American Journal of Clinical Nutrition, Vol. 85, pages 649-650, 2007.

114. Gariballa, British Medical Journal, Vol. 331, pages 304-305, 2005.

115. Lesourd, American Journal Clinical Nutrition, Vol. 66, pages 478s-484s, 1997.

116. Durga and colleagues, Lancet, Vol. 369, pages 208-216, 2007. If you do not subscribe to Lancet, scan down the top page of search engine and you will find the article extracted by other links.

117. Autier, Archives of Internal Medicine, Vol. 167, 1730-1737, 2007 see:

    archinte.ama-assn.org/content/vol167/issue16/index.dtl

118. Whalley, American Journal of Clinical Nutrition, Vol. 87, pages 449-454, 2008.

119. Hsia, Calcium/vitamin D supplementation and cardiovascular events, *Circulation, Vol. 115,* pages 846-854, 2007.

120. Bruno, Free Radical Biology and Medicine, Vol. 40, pages 689-697, 2006.

121. Duara and colleagues, presentation at American Academy Neurology, 60th Anniversary Annual Meeting, Chicago, USA, April 16th, 2008.

122. **www.medscape.com/viewarticle/573383**

123. Thornalley and colleagues, Diabetologia, Vol. 50, pages 2164-2170, 2007.

124. Head and Jurenka, Alternative Medicine Review, Vol. 9, pages 360-401, 2004.

125. Hypponen and Power, Diabetes Care, Vol. 29, pages 2244-2246, 2006.

126. **www.pponline.co.uk/encyc/supplements-athletes.html**

127. **www.food.gov.uk**, and open up "July 2008 EC update on vitamins and minerals in food".

Additional Useful References on Vitamins

128. The British Menopause Society: Fact Sheets. British Menopause Society 4-6 Eton Place, Marlow, Buckingham shire, UK, SL7 2QA. Tel. +44 (0) 1628 890199, Fax: +44 (0) 1628 474042.

129. Wang, and colleagues, present evidence of the benefits of fish oil in cardiovascular disease. American Journal of Clinical Nutrition, Vol. 84, pages 5-17, 2006.

130. Lavie and colleagues, present mounting evidence for fish oils not only preventing heart disease but also reducing mortalities in patients with heart disease. Journal of American College of Cardiology, Vol. 54, pages 585-594, 2009.

131. Dijkstra and colleagues, cast some doubt on benefits of fish oils. European Journal of Heart Failure, Vol. 11, pages 922-928, 2009.

132. The American Journal of Clinical Nutrition –very useful specialist information on latest research on Vitamins: **www.ajcn.org**

133. **www.medicinenet.com** is very useful for information on vitamins.

www.ingramcontent.com/pod-product-compliance
Lightning Source LLC
Chambersburg PA
CBHW050131280326
41933CB00010B/1328